LIVING LIFE IN FAST FORWARD

WHAT CANCER TAUGHT ME ABOUT MAKING TIME COUNT

LIVING LIFE IN FAST FORWARD

WHAT CANCER TAUGHT ME ABOUT MAKING TIME COUNT

JAMES J. HAMMOND

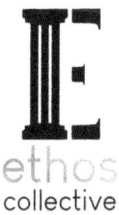

ethos
collective

Living Life in Fast Forward © 2024 by Amanda Hammond Gray

Proceeds from the sale of this book support
research into childhood sarcoma.
www.JJHFund.org

Printed in the United States of America

Published by Ethos Collective™
PO Box 43, Powell, OH 43065
EthosCollective.vip

This book contains material protected under international and federal copyright laws and treaties. Any unauthorized reprint or use of this material is prohibited. No part of this book may be reproduced or transmitted in any form or by any means, electronic or mechanical, including photocopying, recording, or by any information storage and retrieval system, without express written permission from the author.

LCCN: 2024909676
Paperback ISBN: 978-1-63680-295-4
Hardcover ISBN: 978-1-63680-296-1
e-book ISBN: 978-1-63680-297-8

Available in paperback, hardcover, e-book, and audiobook.

Any Internet addresses (websites, blogs, etc.) and telephone numbers printed in this book are offered as a resource. They are not intended in any way to be or imply an endorsement by Ethos Collective™, nor does Ethos Collective™ vouch for the content of these sites and numbers for the life of this book.

Some names and identifying details may have been changed to protect the privacy of individuals.

Table of Contents

Prologue vii
A Note From James. ix
Acknowledgments. xiii
Chapter 1: Fast Forward for Real 1
Chapter 2: Resetting Your Priorities. 7
Chapter 3: Appreciating Life 17
Chapter 4: Choosing Your Attitude 25
Chapter 5: Developing Empathy 35
Chapter 6: Caring for Yourself 45
Chapter 7: Finding Your Purpose 57
Chapter 8: Accepting Support 63
Chapter 9: Conclusion 69
Epilogue 75
Meet James Hammond 77
Credits and Book Recommendations 79

Prologue

I met James Hammond at the beginning of ninth grade. From the moment I laid eyes on him, I had a *little* crush on the cute quarterback. Just friends at first, it took us three years to decide to start dating. As teens head over heels in love, we did everything together. After prom and high school graduation, we decided to go to the same university, move in together, and adopt our Bernese Mountain Dog puppy, Harvin.

Four years later, we graduated from Western University, moved to Toronto, Ontario, bought our first home together, and were married on a beautiful summer day, surrounded by 165 of our closest friends and loved ones. Two weeks following the wedding, James and I loaded our car with our dog and other essentials and headed for our next adventure in San Francisco. We lived in beautiful Northern California for a year and a half, then returned to Toronto in December, only to receive James's first cancer diagnosis three months later.

When James said he wanted to write a book, I was not surprised. Although we joked about the irony of a high school English teacher marrying someone who read his first book in twelfth grade (*A Clockwork Orange* by Anthony Burgess, no less), James's goal of becoming the author of his journey seemed perfectly in character to me. James always had big goals and an even bigger work ethic, and I knew he would make it a reality.

As James's wife, I am, of course, his biggest fan. Even so, I think this book, a collection of life lessons from someone whose life got sped up, has something to offer *most* people. I hope you find the insights James shares in this book to be helpful in your life and in the lives of the people you love.

Amanda Hammond Gray

A Note From James

As the subtitle, "What Cancer Taught Me About Making Time Count," suggests, I hope to use this book to provide you with perspectives, regardless of your circumstances, to substantially improve your life. My cancer, a rare form of pediatric sarcoma, metastasized broadly throughout my body after my physicians thought it had been eradicated, had a significant impact on my perspectives. It compressed my life and brought what mattered into extreme focus.

Although my cancer diagnosis was initially devastating, surprisingly for me, silver linings began emerging from the fog of trauma. I started to consider previously neglected aspects of my life more seriously from a completely new vantage point. Many of these silver linings occurred between my ears. Inside my brain, with all of its oddities and idiosyncrasies, I recognized how my priorities, my attitudes, what I was grateful for, and my life choices were affecting myself and others. With a hint of frustration, I realized I could have appreciated many of these things without enduring so much of the trauma; however, I believe I likely would have never gone through this discovery process otherwise.

The topics for *Living Life in Fast Forward* were largely established from what became most important for me post-diagnosis, as I evaluated my remaining life and what I believed might be the most informative and helpful ideas to share with others. The circumstances leading up to this book forced my eyes open to many of these topics and let me view them with new depth and clarity. I also shared the wisdom of some great minds that have influenced me and shaped my own thinking on these matters. The quotations at the beginning of each chapter have truly resonated with me. I hope you—without having to endure a similar trauma—can take genuine value and perspective from the chapters that follow. I want to help you consider ideas like prioritization, attitude, self-care, empathy, and appreciation without enduring a terminal cancer diagnosis like the one that led me to these perspectives.

As I have tried to do with my own life post-diagnosis, I have limited this book to a small number of focused themes, which make up the eight chapters of *Living Life in Fast Forward*.

While I remain hopeful that we may one day find a cure to eradicate my disease, I continue to be wholly realistic about my incredibly poor odds and cognizant of the way I want to live my life in light of those odds. I am grateful for this opportunity to share my perspectives in my own words. Facing death and uncertainty motivated me to write with the hope of providing you new perspectives—a bit of good that came from my relatively dark times. I encourage you to think deeply about the topics discussed in this book, and I hope it challenges you to act now while you read rather than after a traumatic event forces this thinking on you.

As a reminder, we are in the *living* business, not the *dying* business.

Life is experienced from multiple perspectives—including different ages and maturities, as well as different places psychologically, through both joy and suffering. I needed to experience serious upheaval and face my impending mortality to take a conscious look at life from every perspective. I am confident, however, that a similarly traumatic ordeal is not required to learn through this discovery process.

    I sincerely hope you will take advantage of my somewhat unique perspective and, as you briefly shift your own thinking into fast forward, develop an even greater appreciation for your life, your priorities, and your responsibilities. May every word you read be beneficial to your life and the lives of the ones you love.

Acknowledgments

To my wife, Amanda:
    I have often said throughout this process that it is easier—particularly emotionally—to be the patient than it is to be the patient's spouse, and I very genuinely believe that. Throughout the entire process, I have had a job to do, and I have received so much applause, praise, and support along the way. My wife, Amanda, deserves so much of that praise. I am forever grateful, especially for her emotional strength and toughness, and especially for that strength and toughness when I was not at my best.

To my Parents, Richard and Jo-Anne Hammond:
    Just about everything worthwhile and good I've ever done is owed to them.

To my amazing physicians, Dr. Allan Detsky, Dr. Abha Gupta, and Dr. Pamela Mosher:
    Their exceptional care and support have given me the confidence to keep fighting.

To my army of friends—they know who they are:
    Without them beside me each step of the way, I would never have come so far.

1

Fast Forward for Real

I have realities in my past, not only the reality of work done and love loved, but of suffering bravely suffered. These sufferings are even the things of which I am most proud, though these are things which cannot inspire envy.

—Viktor Frankl

When diagnosed with a terminal illness, your life and the lives of your immediate family change in an instant. A myriad of new challenges hit you. How should you spend your remaining time with family and friends? What should you tell your children? If you don't have kids, should you consider having them? Should you prioritize your work or quit your job and live out your days how you choose to? How should you handle your finances to ensure you don't leave your family with a tremendous burden? What do you need to do to mentally and emotionally process all of the information being thrown at you, be brave, and face your mortality with grace? At the same time, how can you emotionally support your loved ones? How can you retain the right amount of positivity and hope for an unexpected cure yet not disappoint yourself and others as your condition worsens?

I cannot properly explain what it is like to be told that you have cancer, how it feels to have tumors all over your body and know there are countless more inside you, and know you have a very short time to live. In some ways, it is all a little less terrible than you would think. In other ways, it is probably worse.

On the one hand, I had a wonderful life prior to my cancer diagnosis and recurrence—an extraordinary wife, a loving family, fantastic friends, a well-respected and lucrative job, a beautiful home, and hobbies I genuinely loved, like reading, personal fitness, and golf. Being aware of and grateful for this wonderful life made my prognosis easier to swallow. I knew that I had experienced so much love and joy. On the other hand, I was not ready to stop living that beautiful life, so being aware of what I was about to lose made my prognosis feel more harsh and unbearable. Also, seeing the effects of the diagnosis on the faces of my closest friends and loved ones made it clear to me how devastated they were going to be when I did pass away.

My circumstances will sound dark and traumatic, but this entire experience has also been enlightening. Even if all I get is twenty-nine years, I still think I have lived one of the best lives imaginable. I feel tremendously lucky to have experienced all I have and loved all I have loved. Now, I treat each additional day as an unexpected treasure, knowing my life has been permanently set to fast forward. I try to live every day like it is my last while keeping a little bit of hope for an unexpected, emergent cure if I survive long enough to see one. Most importantly, I am now more grateful for each moment than I have been at any other point in my life.

Diagnosis, Treatment, and Recovery

Though I did not realize it at the time, a preliminary diagnosis put my life on fast forward at age twenty-six. The pathologists completed their review of my biopsied tissue, and I was diagnosed with Alveolar Rhabdomyosarcoma (A-RMS), a rare and often lethal form of pediatric sarcoma.

Fortunately, the doctors obtained negative results from the surgically removed right armpit lymph nodes. And in the CT scans of my chest, abdomen, and pelvis, the disease appeared to be localized to a tennis-ball-sized tumor in my dominant right forearm. Although assumed to be localized and treatable, my cancer still represented a big risk. Not only was the cancer pill hard to swallow with the associated lifestyle changes, but it was also nerve-wracking to know that if even a few cancer cells slipped out of my tumor and began to metastasize, I would likely die. For the time being, this scenario appeared to be avoidable, and it looked like, with the help of my tremendous medical and support teams, I could beat this cancer.

For the next nine months, my physicians and I moved through a well-executed plan that included twelve rounds of chemotherapy, twenty-five sessions of radiation therapy (starting after my second round of chemo), and a half-day surgery on my right forearm (after my eighth round of chemo). As frightening as the idea of chemotherapy is, the three-week cycle of treatments became surprisingly routine. The first week involved daily trips to the hospital to receive the intravenous medications that took an hour or two to administer. Thanks to my support team of family and friends, I never had to do this alone. Though I have expressed my gratitude to each of them, they will never truly realize how much the time they spent meant to me. Their presence increased my ability to persevere as the weeks wore on, and the consequences of the treatment took their toll. The second week of each cycle became the worst, with fatigue and nausea almost unbearable, requiring even more medications to combat their effects. By the third week of the cycle, my coping abilities were improving, and I started to feel more myself, only to prepare to repeat the process.

Radiation treatments were interspersed between cycles, with time added to allow my body to recover before beginning chemotherapy again. These treatments involved placing my arm in a mesh cast so it remained perfectly still while the invisible rays did their work. Gradually, I could feel these sessions sapping my energy and requiring more time to recover.

Surgery became the next milestone and a sign that my medical team had confidence the other treatments were working. Because this involved removing most of one muscle in my right forearm, I worried how the surgery would affect my use of it. As I woke up from surgery, I immediately started testing my abilities. Thankfully, I had complete use of my arm, hand, and fingers—which I displayed to my wife by giving her a thumbs-up.

After six months of treatment, the pathologists reviewed my tissue and found no sign of cancer. Tentatively deemed cancer-free, I completed the final four rounds of chemotherapy, primarily as an additional precaution in light of the serious and relentless nature of A-RMS.

I emerged from this process largely unbroken mentally and physically. Only a few physical and emotional scars remained. Thrilled to finish this chapter, yet cognizant of the potential of recurrence, particularly within the first year, I focused on getting back to my normal life and living it as fully as possible. I actively chose not to think about the potential recurrence, reserving my worry for my quarterly check-ups and allowing them to identify any emergent problems.

In my first cancer fight, with the power of an extensive support system, caring and capable physicians and nurses, and an uncompromising focus on staying positive and winning one day at a time, I was able to tolerate the ups and downs of treatment well. Unfortunately, the war was not yet won.

The Recurrence

For five months, I returned to the normalcy of hard work, exercise, eating well, and quality time with family and friends. Then, about two weeks before my twenty-eighth birthday, doctors informed me my cancer had returned and spread throughout much of my body. Though well aware recurrence was possible, my family and I were not prepared. Nor were we ready for how severe the problem now was. Doctors told us they believed the cancer had spread during my first round of treatments at levels too small to detect.

A couple of days later, my caring and brilliant oncologist told my wife and me, through tears, that this time my cancer was incurable. The A-RMS was going to take my life and do so quite quickly. At the time, metastatic A-RMS meant certain death unless an emergent cure presented itself.

After receiving my updated prognosis, my wife and I struggled to compartmentalize my sickness and our day-to-day lives. It weighed on us, particularly on her, constantly. Even activities that normally brought us joy, like going for long walks in our lovely neighborhood or watching one of our favorite TV shows, felt heavy. We would get stuck wondering how many more of these moments we would get before I died. Thankfully, we realized pretty quickly these feelings were unproductive and unsustainable, and we began to regroup and regain our perspective. Our big, happy-go-lucky Bernese Mountain Dog, Harvin, greatly assisted us in this journey.

The Fight

Over the next six months, I completed eight cycles of chemotherapy—seven cycles before my cancer overcame the first regimen and one cycle before my cancer overcame the second regimen. Like my first course of treatments, each cycle consisted of one week of daily intravenous treatments, one week of managing the consequences, and one week of recovery.

Once my team and I realized the chemotherapies were not helping, we decided to address the excruciating pain from my cancer with radiation therapy. The A-RMS deeply penetrated various bones in my leg, hip, back, and shoulder and included an especially dangerous tumor just below my right eye and optical nerve. After a short washout period post-radiation, during which I received no treatment, I elected to participate in a clinical trial at the National Institutes of Health in Bethesda, Maryland, as a way to hopefully regain some control over the disease. This involved monthly trips for tests and treatment, always in the company of one of my wonderful supporters. I knew this was my last hope for recovery, but with no progress after three months, I withdrew. Back with my medical team in Toronto, we are treating the main issues of pain in my back and fluid in my lungs as best we can.

If you think about it, each of our lives will eventually be put into fast forward, even if not to the extreme of my own. I learned many lessons and gained insights and perspective as I journeyed through these past couple of years—lessons I hope will inspire and encourage you, and ones I hope you learn from my trauma rather than facing this degree of Life in Fast Forward yourself.

2

Resetting Your Priorities

Always make your future bigger than your past.

—Dan Sullivan

Ever since I was a child, I fell squarely into the "life is too short" camp. I hated wasting time—things like waiting in long lines, putting away dishes, or even taking the time to dress in warm clothes before heading outside in the winter. I think I had the general sentiment mostly correct: life was not meant to be squandered. Now, on the other side of a terminal diagnosis, my view that life is incredibly short and precious is far stronger and more deeply rooted. I now thoroughly believe life is too precious to spend much time on tasks that do not either fulfill your purpose or bring you joy. What gives people purpose or brings them joy will, of course, vary greatly from person to person, and the process of prioritizing these items is intensely individualized. However, we can all benefit from thinking about our choices and prioritizing through this purpose-joy lens.

Today, many things bring me great purpose and joy, including spending time with my family and friends, traveling and experiencing nature, reading and writing, maintaining my physical fitness, and providing emotional support to others.

You can use this purpose-joy idea to help prioritize the most important events and tasks in your life. The topics in this chapter quickly came to mind when I faced my own thoughts about life and death, but these ideas are valuable focusing tools for any moment in your life.

One of my key insights from Living Life in Fast Forward came from the tension between choosing what to prioritize—and accomplishing those important goals—and wholly enjoying and cherishing each moment, one by one. This dynamic, while challenging, is incredibly rewarding and worth the hard work of thoughtful pursuit. I encourage you to stay mindful of this friction as you apply it to your own life.

Understanding what brings joy and purpose takes self-reflection and self-knowledge. There is a difference between something new or shiny that delivers a brief moment of joy or dopamine and something great or timeless that has a deeper and more meaningful impact on your soul. It could be the subtle difference between something that *has* a purpose and something that *gives* you purpose.

Before I received my diagnosis, one of my goals was to buy a cottage. This was something I looked forward to sharing with my family and truly believed would bring us joy. I made this dream a priority by working long hours and prioritizing my financial goals. Post-diagnosis, this priority shifted. Even if I could beat this disease and live long enough to be able to make this purchase, it no longer interested me if it meant I had to continue with eighty-hour work weeks. Spending time with my family and friends in my twenties and thirties was my new priority.

Questions to Ponder as You Shift to Fast Forward:

- What brings you purpose or joy?
- How can you make these things greater priorities in your life?

Pulling Forward What's Most Important

Naturally, we all have different short-, medium-, and long-term priorities. These priorities may include things like finding a life partner, buying a home, having children, achieving career success and financial security, or traveling the world.

Think about which items from life's long road you would prioritize. Also, consider how you would do so if you only had one, two, or five years to live.

While I would not wish my prognosis on anyone, I am grateful it forced me to look at my life and priorities from this shortened perspective. I recognized having children sooner genuinely mattered to me. I wanted to explore and travel as much as my treatment would allow and spend more time reading and writing, enjoying my wife, family, and closest friends, and doing my best to ensure my family's financial security.

This process also helped me to deprioritize a number of more fickle and materialistic items from further down life's road. These things fall away quickly when your health gets called into question. In the box below are some of the priorities I considered and reassessed, as well as questions you might ask yourself if you want to shift into fast forward.

- Friends and Family – Do you spend enough time with the people you love? Do the people in your life bring you joy?
- Children – Do you want a family? How can you be proud of the parent you are?
- Hobbies (e.g., traveling, reading, writing) – What do you spend your free time doing? Do these things bring you joy?
- Finances – Are you saving for retirement? For a rainy day? Are you making financial choices that will support your family?
- Physical Fitness – Are you prioritizing your physical health? Do you dedicate time to healing and nourishing your body?

My personal and updated list of priorities helped bring direction and happiness—both in the journey of undertaking and in the destination of accomplishing them. I have found the most purpose and joy when I have been able to stay present and surrender to these experiences fully.

Questions to Ponder as You Shift to Fast Forward:

- What specific priorities are most important to you?
- When do you think it makes sense to prioritize each of these things?
- Do any of your former priorities fall away when viewed through this fast-forward lens?
- Does your remaining list feel more suitable?

Turning Longer-Term Thinking into Shorter-Term Goals

I believe that long-term thinking and delayed gratification, rather than short-term thinking and immediate satisfaction, are valuable tools for living a better life. For me, examples of long-term decisions included building strong academic and mental foundations to excel personally and professionally, exercising and eating well to maintain long-term health and increase longevity, investing meaningful time and energy in children so they become upstanding adolescents and adults, and working hard while setting aside money from each paycheck for that inevitable rainy day.

The value of a long-term orientation remains even when you face a terminal illness and a shortened lifespan. However, many of my logical, long-term decisions now depend on who will benefit from the returns. As a result, I found myself seeking intersections between what makes sense for the long-term future and what I can actually accomplish in the short term. For example, spending time with people whose company I cherish is something I enjoy in the present and will, hopefully, have long-term returns for my counterparts. Eating wholesome and nutritious meals and exercising in ways I enjoy (or at least do not dislike) helps me feel better now while also improving my remaining lifetime.

This approach can result in a more rewarding and healthier way of living life—one that can be more fun, more encouraging, and provide you with greater momentum versus focusing exclusively on the long-term future. By taking this perspective, you remain aware of the unattractiveness of taking shortcuts while being realistic and empathetic to your and your loved ones' near-term needs. Importantly, it also translates your long-term decisions and goals into a series of meaningful steps.

While opportunities do exist to marry near- and long-term aspirations, you will no doubt be faced with many situations where you have less freedom to solve both sides of the equation. Applying a slightly different filter in these situations can help simplify your life. Think about how a long-term decision will affect your family, close friends, or your community. If you are confident that your decision will benefit many of these people, your decision is very likely worth making. Such a decision may also bring you a profound sense of purpose. For me, some of the more obvious things worth prioritizing that fall into the long-term camp include financial planning, updating my will, and taking time to share my perspectives on the challenges my family and friends currently or may one day face.

Questions to Ponder as You Shift to Fast Forward:

- How has delayed gratification and long-term decision-making benefitted you so far?
- What activities could you do that will satisfy both present and long-term goals?

Spending Time with the People Who Matter Most to You

Each person you care deeply about—your spouse, family member, friend, colleague, or mentor—plays a unique and critical role in your life, and you likely play a similarly integral role in theirs. Often, these relationships are based on some combination of unconditional love, guidance and mentorship, shared interests, and mutual respect.

In those closest to me, I appreciate unique wit and wisdom, remarkable listening skills, genuine love and care, and unbridled honesty and authenticity. Knowing how much these characteristics mean in my relationships, I seek to embody these traits myself. I realized that I could contribute to building these long and mutually beneficial relationships instead of simply trying to gain from them.

Life is too precious and valuable to miss opportunities to spend time with the people you love the most; these interactions give us energy and direction. The inverse is also true: we lose momentum by spending significant time with people we do not respect. I have become very aware of time spent with people who constantly complain or who lack perspective. Setting a higher bar for who we decide to spend time with is both sensible and liberating. You may feel selfish doing so, thinking: "Who am I to turn away people who want to spend time with me?" But this one is non-negotiable. You should always feel empowered to decide with whom you spend your valuable time. I would strongly argue that avoiding people you do not respect is more *selfless* than selfish. Avoid disrespect or rudeness; these interactions will almost certainly lack value and depth for both you and them. And remember that work and collegial relationships are important, but very few will be with you when you are ninety.

We are some version of a weighted average of the people we have spent the most time with throughout our lives. Being thoughtful about how the time you spend and who you spend that time with shapes who you ultimately become. Positive changes take time to materialize, but they occur most predictably when approached with deliberate intention. Thoughtfully using interactions with people who matter most to you is the best path on your journey to becoming who you aspire to be.

In life, as in business, time and resource allocation is critical. If you would like to arrive at a certain destination in your life—for example, you would like to be a great parent or to excel in a challenging career—you should spend your time in a way that helps you gradually fulfill these roles. Along the way, life will provide you with many distractions that will make you question your time allocation. You need to use your priorities as a filter for how to spend every minute.

Your spouse, immediate family, and closest friends are likely to be some of the most understanding people when it comes to appreciating, accepting, and accommodating your commitments and priorities. These individuals know you best and are likely to have confidence in your ability to properly prioritize and manage your own life, and they'll respect your choices. However, remember that these relationships are the ones that matter the most to us, and we should foster these bonds with immense care.

Invest in relationships with the people you love and cherish most. Failing to do so is a common blind spot in our fast-paced lives. Make the time for the calls, coffees, lunches, and dinners. Deliberately carve out time for the people that matter. These interactions, of course, take lots of time and energy, but they are imperative for living a meaningful life. If you are not willing to make these investments, your relationships will weaken and ultimately deteriorate. As Clay Christensen said: "You can see the costs of investing, but it's really hard to see the costs of not investing."

Questions to Ponder as You Shift to Fast Forward:

- What traits define the people whose time and companionship you cherish most?
- Who are the people in your life who embody the traits you admire?
- How can you prioritize spending more time with them?
- How much time should you invest in your work versus your family, and should this answer change over time?
- How does the way you invest your time affect your spouse or partner and add to their responsibilities?
- What would you do to get a close lost relationship back?

Pursuing Happiness Productively

Pursuing happiness is often a challenging endeavor in and of itself. What makes one person happy is different than what makes another person happy. What we expect to bring happiness does not always yield the intended result. I believe that happiness is experienced less when completing an activity and more when fully engaging with the activity.

In my experience, part of obtaining genuine happiness is, in whatever you are doing, developing some mastery over the task at hand. For example, I fell in love with golf when I was a youth. Playing with my family on warm summer nights and the fact I love being outdoors might have contributed to my passion. Despite my affection for the sport, I have more fun playing when I hit good shots than when I hit bad ones. One thing I really love about the game, and what makes it different from other sports, is that amateur golfers get to do exactly what the pros do, just far less consistently. We can play the same courses and even hit the same pro-quality shots here and there.

An important part of prioritization as a path to genuine happiness is understanding what you are uniquely capable of achieving and what you are passionate about doing. Part of my enthusiasm for golf came because I had early success with the sport and developed a bit of mastery in some of the basic skills. This made me want to practice and get better. To become excellent at anything, of course, takes dedicated effort. However, the journey towards excellence can still be one filled with joy and satisfaction as you relish each step and witness your progress. Always aim high.

A lot of people cheer for the long shot. A win for the underdog is always surprising and often makes for a good story. I tend to find myself cheering for the favorites. I appreciate those all-time greats—individuals or teams that have developed unparalleled excellence in their profession. I want to strive toward the model of greatness. We should work hard and aspire to be great, not to be lucky.

While there are relatively few productive paths to pursuing happiness, there are, unfortunately, a large number of *unproductive* paths to pursuing happiness. Unproductive pursuits of happiness often share some common characteristics, including short-termism, materialism, and lack of presence. In today's world, with the prevalence of smartphones and social media, more and more people seek out and are addicted to short-term dopamine bursts, such as scrolling through Instagram. These devices and mediums exacerbate personal weaknesses like the "fear of missing out," lemming or copycat behavior, and simply not being present in the current moment. There are, of course, far more nefarious pursuits of happiness that are also highly unproductive, including chasing euphoria and short-term highs through chemical or other means. You can also expect very little happiness over time from doing things like eating terribly unhealthy meals or focusing on financial gain.

I appreciate every moment of happiness I've been able to experience since my diagnosis, but most have come through reprioritizing. Don't wait to set priorities that will enhance your life and the lives of those you love.

Questions to Ponder as You Shift to Fast Forward:

- What kind of activities make you happy?
- In what areas of your life would you say you truly excel?
- Are there any unproductive things in your life that you need to stop doing?

3
Appreciating Life

*Gratitude is not only the greatest of virtues,
but the parent of all others.*

—Cicero

Genuine gratitude is essential and takes regular practice. By being appreciative, you remain steady and grounded. Regularly reminding yourself of all the ways you are fortunate helps maintain perspective and optimism. Even in our darkest moments, we *all* have much to be grateful for.

I am certainly not grateful for my cancer or my terminal prognosis, but I am grateful for the *challenge* I have been given. I am also genuinely grateful for a tremendous number of other things, including my loving wife and family, my wonderful friends, my beautiful home, neighborhood, and community, my brilliant physicians, my supportive colleagues, and my many other freedoms and opportunities. I am especially grateful for my wife, and I feel incredibly fortunate to have her love, support, friendship, and pure effervescence for so long.

Throughout my two cancer fights, I developed a far greater appreciation for my life and its good fortunes. Now, I treat every day as a gift, waking up each morning feeling grateful for another opportunity to be with the people I love and do things I cherish. I choose to remain grateful every day, even when, objectively, there may be much more to be upset about than there is to appreciate. I find myself more aware of the beauty in my surroundings and more appreciative of the ability to see and enjoy it. I try to breathe more deeply and to surrender more completely to life.

Another realization about appreciation, for me, has been the importance of actually expressing that appreciation to others.

Receiving sincere appreciation provides great pride and much-needed confidence, affirmation, and direction. You should make the effort to frequently express your genuine appreciation, especially to the people you love and care most about. The cast and crew in your life thrive on your praise, and providing it is a highly rewarding way to make a tremendous contribution to their lives.

Receiving genuine praise, applause, and encouragement during my first cancer fight gave me tremendous energy and confidence to persevere and, once finished, put the fight behind me. Simple phrases like "You are an inspiration," "Your perseverance is incredible," or "I admire your strength" fueled me when fighting became difficult. Every word of affirmation and appreciation helps and is worth providing. No thought is too small.

I like to run myself through an exercise of appreciation every morning shortly after waking up and again in the late afternoon when I find a quiet moment. These quick sessions energize me and leave me with a renewed appreciation for all the positives in my life, even considering the negatives.

Questions to Ponder as You Shift to Fast Forward:

- Has anyone ever told you how great a job you are doing and how much they appreciate or are inspired by your hard work?
- How have these appreciative comments made you feel?
- When was the last time you thought about what you are genuinely grateful for?
- Take a moment to think about the aspects and people in your life today for whom you are most grateful. How does this kind of thinking make you feel?

Cherishing Family and Friends

Even without a crisis, the people in your life need to be cherished, appreciated, and frequently told how tremendously they contribute to your happiness and overall well-being. When faced with a critical illness, this process occurs a bit more automatically. I find myself more frequently expressing my appreciation and affection to my wife, family members, and friends. Everyone, particularly my wife, stayed beside me every step of the way as my health deteriorated. From countless chemotherapy infusions to sleepless and painful nights to many hospitalizations, I knew someone in my support system would be there. They make it extremely easy for me to be grateful, but now I consciously remind myself to say so. Naturally, your family and friends will adjust their contributions to your life according to what each situation demands, but even in the less traumatic moments, they are making a definitive impact on you by listening, providing advice, mentoring, teaching, and simply spending time with you.

Showing sincere appreciation demonstrates your strength and respect, not your weakness. It also just feels good to see how positively people respond. It is another example of doing something that makes sense both today and for the long term. The recipient of your genuine appreciation feels great today and will not soon forget your praise. People will also appreciate you right back, and they are more likely to go out of their way to try to provide assistance when you need it.

Unfortunately, many people are still largely unappreciative of their good fortune and do not take the time to express the gratitude they do feel. I believe this is a great detriment to everyone involved, particularly to those withholding their gratitude. Looking back, I can see many situations where I put more emphasis on being "right" than on the relationship itself. Pride kept me from seeing my good fortune, and I missed out on the joy showing appreciation brings.

Show your gratitude before it is too late—before a relationship deteriorates or life ends. Express your appreciation and gratitude to your family and friends, and be willing to accept their praise and affection with open arms.

Questions to Ponder as You Shift to Fast Forward:

- How often do you tell the people you love that you love them?
- How often do you tell the people who have made significant contributions to your life about the positive impacts they have had on you?

Appreciating Your Joy and Your Suffering

When you experience the things you most enjoy, do just that and surrender to the experience. Also, do not try desperately holding onto or unnaturally extending the experience. Before you wander on to your next task or activity, pause to appreciate the present moment, which is the only place you can experience genuine joy.

Suffering, while necessarily painful, can also be tremendously valuable. Tragedy and heartbreak, whether experienced directly by you or by others, can help you more fully appreciate the magnitude of your joys by comparison. Being diagnosed with a terminal illness or hearing about someone receiving such a diagnosis can give you a better sense of the broad range of potential human experiences. You become more capable of understanding life's peaks and valleys as a result. Being aware of the potential for really bad stuff helps you remain thankful for the good things in your life. With a better perspective, you can place your positive and negative experiences and feelings into a larger, more thoughtful context. As the hip-hop philosopher Curtis "50 Cent" Jackson said: "Sunny days wouldn't be special if it wasn't for rain. Joy wouldn't feel so good if it wasn't for pain."

Our challenges give us perspective, knowledge, and wisdom about the human experience. Obviously, we should not wish for tragedy in our lives, but when it does come, we need to be ready to take the good with the bad. Do not try to evade your suffering. Stare your challenges down. Keep your mind ready and your eyes open to silver linings and opportunities to grow. Life is highly dynamic, sprinkled with highs and lows. If life was filled entirely with joy or entirely with sorrow, it would lack depth and meaning. How would you know what to appreciate?

I believe being aware and grateful for both joys and sorrows makes us more able to accept the positive and negative aspects of our lives as they emerge.

Questions to Ponder as You Shift to Fast Forward:

- Stop right now and consider: what are you most grateful for?
- How can you let the people involved know how you feel about them?

- What have you learned from the times you have experienced suffering?

Eliminating Your Complaining and Self-Pity

Even if you find yourself faced with a terrible situation, remember that your life and current state of affairs could likely be worse. There is also little doubt someone out there is currently dealing with something more difficult. You may have even dealt with something more terrible in the past.

Over the course of my illnesses, I have had a number of pretty unenviable days—the day I found out I had cancer, the day my oncologist told me the danger of my cancer type, the day a test revealed my cancer had returned and spread throughout my body, and the day the prognosis came that cancer would take my life sooner rather than later. On each of these less-than-ideal days, however, I am confident others faced more pressing challenges—they lost loved ones, endured unfathomable physical and emotional pain, or took their last breath. Someone *always has it* worse than me. I have yet to find a day or a challenge improved by complaining. On each of these days, I put my suffering into perspective by thinking about the range of outcomes in our human experience. Considering what others were going through gave me the ability to more capably face my challenges in stride; complaining about my pain would not make me better off.

Complaining works like frowning—the action itself can make you unhappier. People almost universally use it as a way of delegating responsibility in a given situation or life more generally. The complainer tends not to grumble about what *they* have done; they moan about what *others* have done to them. Complaining demonstrates a lack of perspective, maturity, and experience. From a relationship standpoint, complaining makes you unattractive to new and old friends alike, as well as to potential long-term partners in life and in business. As Marcus Aurelius said: "Take away the complaint, 'I have been harmed,' and the harm is taken away."

Complaining and self-pity go hand-in-hand. There will be times when things are difficult, and life feels pretty unfair or at least unlucky. However, complaining and feeling sorry for yourself will not help. I believe avoiding self-pity and steering clear of a "why me?" attitude are critically important in good health and bad. While dying of ALS—a horrible neurodegenerative disease that steals every ounce of a patient's motor function—Morrie Schwartz observed it would be useful for everyone to set a daily limit of self-pity.

If you have a problem, address it. To deal with challenges, you must first take responsibility for your contributions, big or small. Once the problem is dealt with, put it in the past. If your obstacle is difficult or impossible to resolve—like a critical illness—wallowing and complaining about your misfortune will not help. Personally, doing so would only cheapen the time I have left to appreciate the amazing things I can experience.

Questions to Ponder as You Shift to Fast Forward:

- Has complaining about your circumstances ever improved those negative conditions?
- What obstacles and challenges are you currently facing?
- What role did you have in putting yourself in these situations?
- What can you do to resolve the issues at hand?

4

Choosing Your Attitude

*You must never confuse faith you will prevail in the end—
which you can never afford to lose—
with the discipline to confront the most brutal facts
of your current reality, whatever they might be.*

—James Stockdale

The power of the human mind is truly incredible. The brain can overcome immense obstacles, influence the body, and navigate life's complexities. Fortunately, our attitudes and mindsets are also largely in our control, unlike external events and the actions of others in our lives. We possess the capacity to establish our desired attitude. And staying true to our chosen attitude is terrifically valuable, especially when adversity inevitably hits. The greater our sense of inner peace, the more capable we are of accepting and appropriately dealing with things that happen to us.

The connection between the body and the mind is fundamental and inseparable. Your physical health affects your mental health, and your psychological well-being affects your physiological well-being. If you are facing an illness or physical injury, you are more capable of recovering if you care for your mind as much as your body.

Upon my original diagnosis, I was pretty overwhelmed by the fact I had cancer and needed to endure nine months of chemotherapy as well as radiation and surgery. I focused principally on challenges inherent in the *expected* process, including the significant chemotherapy side effects and physical recovery from surgery and radiation, but I was also cognizant of the *potential* for the treatments to fail to yield their intended results. I stayed positive and optimistic, and I believed if I was going to come out the other side okay, I would need to stomach this protocol in bite-sized pieces. My wife and I called it "winning one day at a time," and we took comfort in the momentum from the large and increasing number of "small wins" we accumulated over the nine-month process.

I learned that I could get through long, brutal stretches, gradually and deliberately, by simply focusing on and overcoming what I was directly facing in each moment. I was able to just "run a little bit every day" and "chip away." I did not need to run the marathon all at once. Before I knew it, I had finished the race.

When my cancer recurred, and I was given my terminal prognosis, my wife and I were again, in the moment, completely devastated. Quite quickly, however, we decided to stay positive and optimistic, control our negative emotions, and enjoy every moment together. We also believed our response to this tragedy—with unwavering positivity and resolve—would help others in our lives to cope more easily and even be inspired to grow and persevere in their own lives.

In these two cancer fights, my attitude has been one of the only things that I have had control over, and it has kept me sane. It really is possible and productive to be positive and hopeful even as challenges appear directly in front of you or on your horizon. Your attitude can help you stand upright independently without the need for a constant barrage of distractions and stimulation from your environment. As the pain and physical symptoms of my illness have increased, focusing on the positive in my life has been essential.

Questions to Ponder as You Shift to Fast Forward:

- In what situations has your positive and resilient attitude given you a sense of control and helped you alleviate challenges?
- How often are you able to preserve your desired attitude despite difficult circumstances?

Using Your Attitude to Set Your Tempo

Your external, physical environment, which you have little control over, greatly impacts your internal, emotional environment, which you do have control over. In my experience, lasting happiness and equanimity are more significantly impacted by what is going on inside you versus what is going on around you.

Your positive attitude is the starting point for everything else, and it can have a constructive and compounding impact on every other aspect of your life. If you first look internally for satisfaction, you will be more ready for the bad and the good when they come. Your *perception* of circumstances, rather than the conditions themselves, determines your well-being. From this solid ground, you can more appropriately withstand suffering and more fully experience joy.

Smile often, regardless of your situation: it instantly makes you and others happier. Stand tall, disregarding your emotions; your stance makes you more confident and courageous. Be accepting of every occurrence; openness makes your highs higher and your lows more bearable.

Questions to Ponder as You Shift to Fast Forward:

- Is there a problem you are experiencing where taking a positive attitude might help?
- How can you present a positive attitude to others?

Responding to Adversity

In life, we do not get to choose our futures. We do, however, get to decide how we will respond to what the future brings. Our circumstances don't make us great; the way we respond defines our characters. For example, responding to adversity with grace, humility, and courage is truly extraordinary.

Everyone has the opportunity to determine how they will respond to hardship. As Viktor Frankl, a holocaust survivor, said: "Forces beyond your control can take away everything you possess except for one thing: your freedom to choose how you will respond to the situation."

No matter the difficulty or misfortune, try to appreciate, with an open mind, the challenge you have been given and the opportunity to grow.

When adversity strikes, it is crucial not to overreact. Instead, rationally process the situation and dissociate your feelings and well-being from the difficulty itself. Happiness and emotional well-being are not determined exclusively by the vacillations of life. As Marcus Aurelius said: "Do not say, 'I am unhappy because this happened to me.' Not so: say, 'I am happy, though this has happened to me.'"

Questions to Ponder as You Shift to Fast Forward:

- How do you think responding positively to adversity affects your chances of overcoming it?

- What impact would doing so have on your success in life?

Overcoming Your Pain and Suffering

Pain can be terrible. Physical pain can be debilitating. It can negatively impact your sleep and prevent you from participating in life. Emotional pain and suffering can be even more devastating. However, recognizing your ability to cope with pain and suffering can be valuable for your personal growth and development despite the challenge.

When possible, pain and suffering should, of course, be avoided. However, you can use unavoidable pain and suffering as a source of growth and development. When you respond to these negative experiences in a healthy and thoughtful way, you learn toughness and bravery. You are not the same person before and after a significant hardship. If handled appropriately, you become a more complete and mature version of your prior self.

I was certainly scarred—physically and emotionally—by the pain and suffering associated with my initial cancer fight. One of the first times I grasped the magnitude of how much I had changed was when I drove by the hospital after completing treatment. During the chemotherapy and radiation, I was fully in the fight and generally less sensitive to the true gravity of the situation as well as the associated mental and physical burden. When I unintentionally drove by the hospital with my health, for the time being, fully restored, I realized my cancer had also left emotional wounds beyond the scars on my body. My first cancer fight taught me about myself, the power of the mind, and the resilience of the human body.

In my second cancer fight, physical pain became a near-constant battle. Once my cancer spread into the bones of my legs, hips, and pelvis, the pain was intense and, at times, debilitating. Your mind has the ability to make your pain and suffering significantly worse. Based on my experience and on the experiences others have shared with me, dreading, running from, wallowing in, extrapolating, or failing to move on from the pain and suffering can amplify it. Dealing with physical or emotional pain directly and rationally can save you a considerable amount of suffering. As Alan Watts said: "Animals feel pain simply and without dread; humans are overshadowed with anxiety… Real suffering doesn't come from any momentary sensitivity to pain but from our marvelous powers of foresight and memory."

A surefire way to increase your suffering is to dread and obsess over future pain—for instance, an upcoming personal confrontation or serious medical procedure. Whether you worry obsessively or not, you must still endure the pain when you get to it. The advanced suffering you put yourself through will not take away any of the actual trauma. Your dread and obsession, in and of itself, ensures suffering even if the object of your stress ends up being quite tolerable. You will save yourself a lot of misery by crossing the bridge when you get there—ready to face pain if it comes but not obsessing over it in advance.

Also on the list of worst things you can do with pain is imagining it will continue forever or assuming because it is worse today than it was yesterday, it will increase daily. The flawed logic adds to your suffering. In reality, your pain and suffering are not likely to last long. Even the most severe and dramatic physical or emotional pain has an expiration date once it has been properly addressed and managed or treated. Look your pain directly in the eyes and move toward dealing with it. Take solace in your history of overcoming challenges so you can be rational about your pain's duration. Wounds heal, and so do you.

A final, dependable way to experience more suffering than required is failing to move on with your life once your pain has passed. After you successfully endure a challenging, potentially terrible event and recover from it, leave it there. It does not need to become part of you and your future.

With all this said, ongoing suffering needs to be addressed. Recovery can be challenging when the healing process is long. In every case, when you make it to the other side of the pain and treatment, you'll discover you have grown as you've overcome the obstacles. You can leave your pain and suffering behind and bring a new perspective into all your tomorrows—a perspective you earned from having conquered something extraordinary.

Properly addressing pain is person-specific, but I believe key principles apply to most incidents of individual suffering. As I think about some of my own emotional distress—for example, knowing I have a short time to live and my wife will be a widow—as well as my physical agony, one of the most helpful tactics has been being fully aware of the pain and not to trying to run from it. When pain is unavoidable, it is no use trying to hide.

I believe pain and suffering—like fear—do their worst, most destructive work in the shadows. There are many tools and resources to help with emotional and physical pain that can be used thoughtfully, but only when you are aware, realistic, clear-eyed, and present about your pain.

Another useful technique for overcoming pain and mental anguish is to remind yourself how strong you can be. Remember the last time you experienced pain and overcame it. If the pain and suffering you face are new and particularly severe or acute, take solace in your prior successes and know that many others have endured similar hardships.

Lastly, I have found extraordinary energy to persevere by thinking about *who* I am really fighting for. I remind myself that if I am able to effectively move through my pain and suffering, I can be a better husband, son, brother, and friend. This belief helps me to overcome even my most severe discomfort.

Questions to Ponder as You Shift to Fast Forward:

- What pain and suffering have you overcome?
- What has changed in you as a result of those experiences?

(Patiently) Waiting for the Future to Unfold

As much as we would like to think otherwise, we have relatively little control over what happens in the present moment and even less authority over the future. The uncertainty can cause anxiety, yet we seem to think about it constantly, and, unfortunately, we tend to concentrate on the less-than-positive versions of the future.

To me, this practice makes little sense. We should accept the fact there are things we cannot change and spend our energy only where we can conceivably change the outcome.

Focus on your current reality. There is little value in allowing your mind to run wild, bouncing around frantically, thinking about a myriad of potential for both positive and negative futures. Like directing your thoughts on future pain and suffering before it happens, dwelling on potentially unfortunate futures, which may or may not materialize, is counterproductive and distressing. The troublesome events you fear will come may, in fact, look dramatically different or not occur at all by the time you eventually get there. While less problematic than obsessing over negative futures, fixating on possible positive futures can also have its downsides. Thinking about any future outcomes for any extended period of time pulls us away from having genuine experiences in the present—experiences we can see, feel, hear, and truly enjoy.

I am not suggesting being blissfully ignorant of potential challenges and opportunities that may emerge in your future. Preparedness is important—both in and of itself and for the confidence and comfort that comes along with it. If you *must* worry about uncertain futures, try to do so in a constructive way by imagining *solutions* to any emergent challenges. I believe the best approach is to patiently wait for the future to come while enjoying the truly valuable moments of the present.

Questions to Ponder as You Shift to Fast Forward:

- How often do you dwell on potential bad outcomes, personally or professionally, like upcoming projects, medical appointments, or dreaded social commitments?
- How often, when you are facing a challenge, do you reflect on your biggest and most pride-inducing successes?

Exhibiting Relentlessness and Perseverance

To me, relentlessness and perseverance are more states of mind than consequences of human skill. I believe they can grow over time with experience—failure as well as success. I also believe it takes a conscious decision to embody these positive qualities. These attributes don't merely happen day after day; still, I see them in people who, particularly in tough situations, find a way to fight and live for something or someone other than themselves. A mindset of relentlessness and perseverance directly impacts a person's ability to demonstrate resilience and determination in the face of any challenge. Like muscles, these skills need exercise.

Sometimes, we need a confidence boost. Taking inventory of everything we have been able to overcome and accomplish is a powerful way to increase confidence and, in turn, increase our relentlessness and perseverance. Knowing I beat cancer once gave me more confidence and hope in my ability to bravely fight cancer for the second time despite its currently incurable nature.

We all have finite amounts of willpower. You should, therefore, limit the number of times you rely exclusively on personal determination to succeed. Design your life in a way that caters to you and your goals.

Questions to Ponder as You Shift to Fast Forward:

- When has relentlessness been important in your life?
- What major obstacles have you overcome in your life so far?

5

Developing Empathy

No one cares how much you know until they know how much you care.

—Theodore Roosevelt

People desperately want to be heard and understood. Accordingly, you can help others, and others can help you, by listening carefully and being compassionate. Empathy, which encompasses understanding, compassion, and sharing the feelings of others, is a remarkable and often underappreciated skill. The virtue is both rewarding to possess and inspiring to see in others. It contrasts with sympathy—feeling pity or condolence for another person. I believe in the power of empathy, not sympathy.

During the course of my two cancer fights, particularly the more recent, terminal one, I developed a greater appreciation for human empathy, both by witnessing others genuinely demonstrate the virtue towards me and by becoming more empathetic myself. I was humbled by how well certain individuals were able to understand, appreciate, and empathize with what I was going through. Constantly cognizant of not wanting to burden my friends and family with the gravity of my situation or to worry them about the state of my health, only a select number of incredible people have been open to every detail I felt comfortable sharing. In return, they listened carefully, provided tremendous compassion, offered ongoing physical and emotional presence, shared my burden, provided ample applause, and even infused some much-needed humor. These people exemplified complete, genuine empathy to my great benefit.

From my own situation, I developed a far greater appreciation and understanding of others' sorrow and pain. I find it particularly hard to watch children going through the sorts of treatments I endured. Although my cancer is pediatric, and I was typically treated with fellow adults, my primary oncologist was split between adults and children. As I observed these young souls bravely fighting rare, complicated, and often terrifying diseases, their courage and attitude inspired me. My oncologist advised me early on, "Think like a kid: they do great because they have no rear-view mirror." Though ultimately unsuccessful for me, the trial provided strength as I witnessed brave children and their families persevere through continuous streams of challenges and unknowns.

You have the power to greatly improve the lives of your friends and loved ones by being attentive and empathetic in times of need. The tremendous value that empathy from compassionate individuals has had on your ability to overcome should encourage you to pass along the kindness.

Questions to Ponder as You Shift to Fast Forward:

- During the times when you have suffered the most, who helped you cope?

- What key characteristics did those people embody in those crucial moments?

Being Compassionate

Every person has their own specific circumstances, challenges, and aspirations. We are all shaped by our histories, future plans, and the key individuals in our lives. Nevertheless, we all benefit from the genuine compassion of others. We *should* want all people to flourish so they can contribute to their families, communities, and the world at large. As the Dalai Lama said, "The essence of compassion is a desire to alleviate the suffering of others and to promote their well-being."

Having positive, compassionate feelings towards others is an important part of living a good and healthy life. It's likely you have people in your life, and hopefully, plenty, for whom you genuinely wish the very best. You sincerely want them to succeed, and when they do, you feel genuine joy. You hope they avoid suffering, so their suffering causes you genuine distress. The greater the number of people who fit into this category, the better. Appreciating your many meaningful relationships fuels your longevity and well-being.

On the other end of the spectrum, you might have people for whom you feel no compassion. You might even downright dislike them. Still, for your own good, you should never wish suffering on that person. Everyone has their own story and idiosyncratic challenges, most of which they keep private; you may not know the whole story behind their situation. Accordingly, be hesitant about judging them too harshly. A judgmental attitude is, at best, unproductive and, at worst, inhumane.

In my fight, I have had so many in my corner—people who desperately wanted my suffering to end and people who dream and pray for my health and well-being to improve. This group includes not only my family and closest friends but also my physicians and an astonishing number of people I barely know. For this reason and many others, I consider myself incredibly lucky despite my terrible disease and prognosis. While these people almost certainly cannot change my fate, their compassion holds me up and gives me immense strength. So, be like them—be compassionate to others and watch them reap the rewards.

Questions to Ponder as You Shift to Fast Forward:

- Are there people in your life who deserve your compassion but do not currently receive it?
- Who would you take a bullet for, and who would take a bullet for you?

Listening to Others and Sharing Their Pain—and Joy

An important early step towards being empathetic is becoming a great listener. You'll find extreme value in listening intently, using eye contact and internal quietness, and never worrying about what you say next in virtually all settings. However, the skill becomes especially useful when you sit with someone who needs your help and support. Be completely present in the moment, confident you will know what to say and what not to say after listening to their full story, with no need to fill up your mind with your own thoughts while they share theirs. Also, make the effort to listen carefully and attentively even when you do not like or agree with some or all of what you hear.

Good listening is virtuous for both the speaker and the listener. For the speaker, listening well makes them feel as if what they say is important. Knowing they are heard and recognizing that the listener cares about them and their perspectives encourages the speaker to share every piece of important information and allows them to get out what they need to. If you're the listener, being attentive allows you to truly understand and interpret what you hear. You can also enjoy the benefit of building a reputation for being a terrific listener, which can be applied in every interpersonal setting.

The most challenging, and potentially the most rewarding, aspect of empathy is sharing others' pain and suffering. When you care deeply about someone, you tend to feel genuine anguish when they experience physical or emotional trauma. Some see this as a downside of empathy because it can take a toll on the empathizer. As such, you should carry the burden of others only to the extent you have the capacity to do so. For me, sharing the weight of others' physical and emotional pain was uplifting when I compared it with actually enduring the suffering.

It's important to note—sharing pain and suffering is *not* about sharing miserable and unproductive thoughts. We should not wallow on another's behalf, just as the person suffering should not. Likewise, we should not carry around dread for others' possible future suffering. Nor should we extrapolate their current pain into the future or fail to move on once the sufferer's pain has ended.

When friends and family feel discomfort or distress and heartache, listening intently plays an important role. Painful memories carry great power. Acting as support for a loved one during these times may have a significant impact on their lives. When the circumstances are reversed, your family and friends can play this critical role for you.

Not all empathy needs to be focused on pain. Taking great joy in happiness and sharing enjoyment may be the easiest and most natural version of empathy. When you genuinely want another person to have a good life, you in share their happiness. As in the pursuit of our own happiness, we should encourage others to remain fully engaged in the process, focused on their improvement or mastery and guided by their unique passions or abilities. Then, we can help them celebrate, embrace, and fully surrender to their joy.

Questions to Ponder as You Shift to Fast Forward:

- Who is the best listener you know?
- What makes them this way?
- How can you become a better listener?

Being Perceptive

I often wonder, "What does a person in my position, or an equally painful situation, need from their family and friends?" I believe family and friends feel bad and struggle with not knowing how they can help. People want to contribute to the suffering person's life, but they get stuck thinking about what that looks like. Even as a person living out this situation, I am not certain what I need from my family and friends. Loved ones, therefore, should certainly not feel bad for not knowing how to positively contribute.

Naturally, each person who goes through a challenging time has different needs. Some people are far better at understanding what they need than others. Most people who suffer truly appreciate others genuinely caring about their well-being and providing them with unconditional support. For example, I had people in my life say, "Let me know what I can help with, and I'll just sit right here and read until you need me." I was also tremendously fortunate to always have someone to be with me during chemotherapy. Their presence made such a difference. Our efforts needn't be complicated or elaborate to be helpful.

Questions to Ponder as You Shift to Fast Forward:

- When has someone truly helped you in a difficult situation?
- How important was simply their presence with you?

Forgiving Others—and Yourself

Unfortunately, life is irreversible. There is no rewind button. If you made mistakes or if others' mistakes have hurt you, it is best to forgive and move on. As Marcus Aurelius said: "Let a wrong that is [done] be left where it was done." In terms of self-forgiveness, we should certainly not give ourselves unlimited free passes for unacceptable behavior. We should, however, give ourselves a pass when we feel genuine remorse and learn to behave more responsibly. Forcing ourselves to relive our past indiscretions is unproductive and potentially harmful to making progress. Your life is already full of challenges. You do not need to make things incrementally more painful by constantly beating yourself up. I have had to forgive myself for working insanely long hours and missing quality time with friends and family. I can never get that time back, but I can make better use of the time I have left.

Displaying resentment for something done to you is an equally worthless act. Holding onto the anger is more likely to hurt you than the offender, who may or may not be aware of your feelings. Harboring bitterness allows a negative event from your history to damage your current situation. Life is far too precious to spend time holding grudges.

Forgiving yourself and others will allow you to move on from negative or painful events and help you avoid wallowing in past mistakes and injustices. Once you have moved on, you can focus on the things in your life that matter most to you. You can benefit tremendously by having a short memory for the bad things that happen in your life. Instead, practice having a long memory for the great things that happen. As Viktor Frankl said, "I do not forget any good deed done to me, and I do not carry a grudge for a bad one."

Questions to Ponder as You Shift to Fast Forward:

- When was the last time you forgave yourself for something?
- Is there anyone you need to forgive now?

Understanding Fairness

A common and justifiable human desire is to be treated fairly. When we are negatively impacted by an unfair outcome, we feel frustrated. On the other hand, if the unfair event impacts us positively, we may feel lucky and as if the result was not deserved.

Intentional unfairness is, of course, unacceptable. At the same time, many unfortunate events get mischaracterized as unfair ones. There is a vast difference between unfair—an intentional wrong—and an unlucky or random turn of events. When we believe something is unfair, we feel wronged or victimized. Self-pity can set in, constraining our ability to persevere. Though just as unpleasant, unlucky situations happen all the time—to both good and bad people. They happen irrespective of character or circumstances. I believe appreciating the difference between luck and fairness is important for our well-being and ability to cope. Just because something is bad does not mean that it is unfair, and there is always a chance we influenced the unpleasant outcome.

Like most, I am more capable of accepting events I view as unfortunate than those I perceive as unfair. I can more readily face the challenge at hand when I believe the source of the problem is bad luck versus an injustice. Neither my critical illness nor my expected mortality can I see as unfair. I do view them as terribly unlucky, tragic, and unexpected.

Most of my friends and family, however, view my situation as extremely unfair, even though I encourage them not to. Nobody deserves to have a critical illness. I just got very unlucky.

With that said, I have had a genuinely wonderful life. Even after my recurrence diagnosis, my life is good, with much to be grateful for. Had I looked at my situation as unfair, I firmly believe I would be less grateful, hopeful, and resilient. A positive perspective will not magically make the bad event go away, but it will increase your capability to process and overcome it effectively.

As a young adult, I lost a close friend to a tragic train accident. Losing him was jarring. At the time, I thought that his death was unfair, but now I see it as extremely bad luck—a complete fluke. This tragedy led another close friend and me to establish a charitable foundation in our friend's name. We wanted to support underprivileged youth athletes, a service our late friend benefitted from growing up. Running the foundation has shown us some unfairness. For example, some parents use disposable income on frivolous expenses and leave too little for their children's sports and extracurriculars. But, for the most part, we get to help families who have simply come on some bad luck or are forced to face unfortunate circumstances.

Life is more *unpredictable* than it is *unfair*. Each person will have their own unique adventure through life. Lucky and unlucky events deserve no special celebration or blame—they are not personal. Take them in stride.

Questions to Ponder as You Shift to Fast Forward:

- How do you feel when you are treated unfairly?
- In what situations do you find unfairness to most frequently be a problem?

6

Caring for Yourself

Treat yourself like someone you are responsible for helping.
—Jordan B. Peterson

Sometimes, the most *selfless* thing to do is simply to take care of yourself—mentally and physically. By taking care of your own mind and body first, you become more capable of taking care of your family and friends. Your skills for identifying and managing your life's most important commitments increase, and you cannot properly help others if you are not at your best. I am not suggesting you run and hide from your commitments or neglect your friends and loved ones to focus on yourself. Instead, I encourage you to invest the additional energy and clarity you obtain from good, regular self-care into managing your relationships. I found that after I had prioritized my own well-being, I had more of myself to pour into my family and friends.

One benefit of self-care is stress reduction. Stress can have a significant impact on various aspects of your life, including temperament, sleep quality, and physical health. You can actually see stress and its impacts on your brain, body, and immune systems. Dr. Gabor Mate calls it the physical-neurological-immune supersystem[1]. The mind and the body are inseparably connected—the mind impacts the body, and the body impacts the mind. As Dr. Mate said, "It is impossible for any stressful stimulus, chronic or acute, to act on only one part of the super-system."

Questions to Ponder as You Shift to Fast Forward:

- In what parts of your life do you need to start putting yourself first?
- What benefits will this have for you and for others?

The Invincible Me

Throughout my entire post-secondary schooling and professional life, until my terminal diagnosis, I operated at virtually full throttle all the time. At first, a substantial portion of my time and energy went to completing two demanding university degrees concurrently in business and in actuarial science while also obtaining an actuarial professional designation.

By the time I started my first summer internship in finance, I ridiculously began planning for the private equity job I hoped to start two years after graduation—a goal I achieved after landing an exceptionally demanding role in investment banking.

Despite the large educational and professional burdens, I also tried to be fully engaged in almost every other part of life—friends, family, my girlfriend-then-fiancé-then-wife, travel, sports, and personal fitness. I tried to do and have

---

1 Mate, Gabor. *When The Body Says No: The Cost of Hidden Stress.* Toronto, ON: Vintage Canada. 2004.

everything. I did sacrifice varsity sports for my academics, but I was otherwise unrelenting in my need to keep all my other personal balls in the air while juggling the educational and professional ones as well.

For example, in my fourth year of university, I was enrolled in seven business and actuarial science courses, versus the usual five, studying for my fourth Society of Actuaries professional exam (for which the SOA recommends 300 hours of study time) and playing intramural sports, while spending as much time as possible time with friends and family. Looking back, I realize my sleep habits, work hours, stress levels, downtime, and relaxation were terrible.

Some of my overachieving was driven by pride, overconfidence, and ignorance. I liked knowing that relatively few people could or were willing to do what I was doing. I foolishly assumed I needed less sleep than most people and, equally irrationally, that I was somehow invincible.

My shift in focus began gradually with my original cancer diagnosis. However, virtually overnight, with my terminal cancer diagnosis a year later, I started to appreciate the value of deliberate and thoughtful self-care. While neither I nor my physicians believe my hectic schedule caused my cancer, I do wish I had focused more on my own overall well-being prior to my diagnosis. From my original diagnosis onwards, I have seen the significant impact of effective self-care on my well-being, especially when times get particularly tough.

Self-care is a virtuous cycle. Any positive change to your well-being is an achievement in and of itself, and, excitingly, that positive change will likely lead to additional positive changes, which will also likely lead to even more positive changes. Taking deliberate, small steps to improve yourself can have incredibly positive, long-term changes. As Eric Greitens said, "Great changes come when we make small adjustments with great conviction… While real transition does occur in someone's life, it usually happens through evolution, not revolution."

Questions to Ponder as You Shift to Fast Forward:

- When have you been most capable of helping friends and family members through challenging situations?
- When have you been most clearsighted, levelheaded, and thoughtful?
- Is stress impacting your happiness, mood, sleep, or general health?

Establishing Unbreakable Rules and Principles and Following Them

Creating and following rules for yourself can help you to live the fullest life possible. Your rules and principles can give you momentum as you evolve into the person you want to be. Establishing a rules-based lifestyle can also save you time and energy because your rules will help you quickly and automatically deal with little daily questions or challenges. For example, "Should I put my dishes and laundry away?" "Should I make my bed after I wake in the morning?" "Should I donate to the charity that just knocked on my door?" "Should I drink this second (or third or fourth) cup of coffee today?" All these little decisions, without rules and principles, can take up a tremendous amount of your precious mental energy. Your rules and principles can automate decisions for you. By establishing built-in responses to these and many other daily problems, you can greatly simplify your life.

When you do face more complex questions, like dealing with tragedy or loss, making a career move, adapting to an uncomfortable new environment, or solving a challenging personal or professional problem, you will have more time and energy to dedicate yourself fully to the most important and demanding aspects of your life.

For simplicity, my rules start with either *"I will always…"* or *"I will never…"* They include high-level principles, like always being trustworthy, open-minded to new ideas, dedicated to family and friends, focused on living one day at a time and keeping my word, as well as never inflicting pain on any person or animal or making anyone feel stupid. I also have specific principles for day-to-day activities, like always using someone's name, thanking people sincerely, dedicating time to read every day, and looking people in their eyes when they speak. Additionally, I maintain firm rules for sleep, exercise, diet, and mindfulness. Prior to my recurrence, I would tend to revisit my rules every quarter to make sure they remained relevant.

You can, over time, change dramatically for the better when you are deliberate and focused on the right principles. Rules help you become a better version of yourself—bit by bit and day by day. The resulting habits make your life more straightforward and enjoyable.

To benefit from a principles-based lifestyle, however, you must *follow* the rules you establish. Doing so takes self-discipline and moral strength. Clay Christensen says that your personal moral line is only powerful because you do not cross it, and once you justify crossing it once, there is no stopping you from doing it again.

Questions to Ponder as You Shift to Fast Forward:

- Have you created "I will always…" and "I will never…" lists for yourself?

Prioritizing Exercise and Nutrition

I strongly believe in the power of nutrition and exercise to improve mental and physical health and increase resilience.

Your body and mind need fuel to perform at their best. Good, healthy exercise and nutrition habits, like rigorous daily activity and eating wholesome, nourishing foods, energize your body and mind and help you avoid many irritating and unnecessary illnesses and injuries. Taking these simple, daily steps is one of the highest return-on-investment choices you can make. For example, the Canadian Medical Association Journal noted: "Physical inactivity is a modifiable risk factor for cardiovascular disease and a widening variety of other chronic diseases... Men and women who reported increased levels of physical activity and fitness were found to have reductions in relative risk (by about 20%-35%) of death."[2] Dealing with the repercussions of poor exercise and nutrition, such as obesity, heart disease, and diabetes, can be painful and costly. As Benjamin Franklin said: "An ounce of prevention is worth a pound of cure."

Partway through my initial cancer fight, I stopped eating meat and dairy and reduced my refined sugar intake. Throughout my initial fight, I also prioritized regular cardiovascular exercise whenever my nausea and fatigue allowed. I found this approach provided me with significant energy and established, within each round of chemotherapy, a virtuous cycle whereby exercising and eating well made me feel more energetic and lively. As an added bonus, it allowed me to be better able to exercise and eat well the next day. While this is my preferred method, you should select the nutrition and exercise regimen that best fits your own body and needs. Whatever you choose, being and looking healthier will increase your happiness.

Did you know you should drink fluids before you become thirsty? Thirst is your body's way of letting you know you are

---

[2] *National Library of Medicine.* "Health Benefits of Physical Activity: the Evidence. March 14, 2006. https://www.ncbi. nlm.nih.gov/pmc/articles/PMC1402378/.

already dehydrated. In the same way, you should prioritize your health and nutrition before a serious illness or injury forces you to.

Questions to Ponder as You Shift to Fast Forward:

- How could you improve your exercise and eating habits?
- What is one habit that is most important to change?

Allocating Time to Sleep and Restoration

Sleep has become widely recognized as critically important to our health. Many books and reference materials do a good job describing this topic, particularly *Why We Sleep* by Matthew Walker. These resources highlight good sleep hygiene practices like limiting caffeine, exercising regularly, getting vitamin D, and minimizing alcohol and screen time, especially near bedtime. The health benefits of sleep are immense: longer life expectancy, enhanced memory, greater creativity, weight loss, greater resilience, more energy, and lowered risk of heart attack, stroke, and diabetes. You also look and feel better when you are well-rested.

Our bodies know what we need. We just need to listen to them. When we prioritize and understand the importance of sleep, we will discover the amount our individual body requires. Allocating enough time for a peaceful time of rest is vital.

Being diagnosed with cancer was a good wake-up call for me. Prior to that time, I viewed sleep as important and enjoyable but nothing to be given precedence over work or personal commitments. Working eighty-plus hours each week and trying to juggle personal commitments left no time to create deliberate sleeping practices. I frequently slept less than four or five hours a night and lived that way for over five years. Doing so not only negatively impacted my cognitive ability but also damaged my emotional and physical well-being. I potentially exposed myself to serious medical issues, something "invincible" twenty-somethings rarely consider.

During my second cancer fight, I struggled with severe sleep deprivation. My large and numerous tumors made it nearly impossible to find a sleeping position that did not cause serious discomfort. Many of these sleeping positions also exacerbated my cancer-related bone and pancreas pain. I saw the vicious feedback loop of getting inadequate sleep. Each day, my energy level decreased as my pain level increased.

You are not yourself when you are sleep-deprived. You are less resilient, and you are weaker and less capable than your rested self. By not sleeping enough and taking on too much stress, I may have given my cancer an easier opportunity to attack my body.

Questions to Ponder as You Shift to Fast Forward:

- How much longer would you sleep if someone could handle your late-night or early-morning commitments?
- When would you wake up if you did not set an alarm?

Prioritizing Meditation and Reflection

Relaxation techniques, such as the various forms of meditation and yoga, have been shown to have measurable health benefits. While some individuals continue to be uncomfortable with the practice, adopters have benefitted greatly in terms of lower blood pressure, increased cortical activity, and decreased stress, along with many second-order benefits. Take time each day and each week to allow yourself to unwind, understanding that doing so will look different for you than others. The human mind requires stimulation as well as time to rest, process, and reconfigure. Being more reflective, more comfortable with your own mind, and more at peace regardless of your surroundings directly benefits your happiness and overall health. The goal is to be more in control of your own emotions and, as Sam Harris said, "to be happy before anything happens, before one's desires are gratified, in spite of life's difficulties, in the very midst of physical pain, old age, disease, and death."

When I started dipping my toes into meditation and relaxation techniques, I was quite skeptical about how beneficial it would be for me. I was also concerned I would not be good at meditation, given my mind was so infrequently at rest. For example, for a number of years before and during university, it took me at least an hour to fall asleep each night—my mind raced wildly even though my body was exhausted. Today, I could not live without meditation and structured relaxation. I enjoy highly rewarding methods of unwinding, which include daily meditation, yoga and stretching, outdoor walks and runs, and conversations with close friends. I had experimented with meditation previously; however, it was only after receiving my terminal diagnosis that I began meditating more deliberately. For two fifteen-minute periods each day, I use the quite straightforward *Z Technique*[3], which includes mindfulness (present), meditation (past), and manifesting (future) components. I think of this time as two micro-vacations each day—ones I benefit from greatly. Not only do I experience greater calmness and acceptance, but I also feel additional energy and wakefulness after each session. This extra vitality has been a pleasant surprise in coping with chemotherapy-associated chronic fatigue.

While this particular approach has worked well for me, there are many other techniques that are likely to work well for you. Take time to assess each alternative based on your

---

[3] Fletcher, Emily. *Stress Less Accomplish More: Meditation for Extraordinary Performance.* New York, NY: William Morrow. 2019.

own needs and criteria. Importantly, if you select a meditation practice, focus on adherence to the practice as opposed to mastery over it.

Meditation is a subjective exercise, and you will naturally improve over time, but not necessarily in even increments. You should feel confident you will obtain the *benefits* of meditation long before you develop excellence in the practice. The goal of meditation and reflection practices should be to continually, over time, make your mind more healthy.

Questions to Ponder as You Shift to Fast Forward:

- How often do you take time to consciously relax?
- How might daily meditation help you?

Eliminating Excuses for You and Your Loved Ones

A healthy mind accepts responsibility for its actions and its role in a situation. The inverse of taking responsibility is making excuses for yourself or for others. Excuses merely comfort us short-term. They will not allow us to fix behaviors that caused problems in the first place, and they remove every opportunity to challenge ourselves to improve or grow. Instead, they symbolize wiping our hands clean of any responsibility and assigning blame to external things, events, or people.

Similarly, making excuses for loved ones robs them of the freedom to better themselves. By refusing to let them off the hook, we allow them to do the hard work of accepting and learning from their mistakes. There is little benefit to taking it too easy on the people we care about. Of course, you still need to be empathetic and respectful. We don't help others when we provide justification for not accomplishing their goals. They will one day face a situation where no excuse can rescue them. Help them be ready to face the consequences.

Questions to Ponder as You Shift to Fast Forward:

- How often do you make excuses for yourself? Some common ones are "life just got in the way" or "I am so busy."
- How frequently do you provide excuses for other people? For instance, "There is no way you could have known" or "You just have so many things on your plate."

7
Finding Your Purpose

If something's the thing to do, you do it.

—Warren Buffett

Figuring out what you do best—professionally and personally—greatly impacts your quality of life. What fills your schedule fills your mind, and what fills your mind determines who you become.

Finding your purpose is tricky and often takes trial and error. The fear of choosing wrong can lead to making no choice at all, so you have to start somewhere. After you find your purpose, you may realize you are not currently fulfilling it, resulting in significant expenses if you have to make big changes. It is best to recognize those costs as valuable investments.

Prior to my initial cancer diagnosis, I had been very good at living out *other peoples'* dreams. This dynamic was due, in part, to my competitiveness but in larger part to my lack of genuine, introspective thought regarding *my own* dreams. For example, in university, I was accepted into a coveted business administration program. Once there, I earned some of the highest grades, obtained two of the most "sought-after" finance internships, and then, upon graduation, worked at one of the top investment banks. I also received my actuarial professional designation prior to graduation, something my actuarial science classmates wanted desperately.

Shortly after joining the investment bank, I received an offer to join an extremely respected private equity firm eighteen months before the job would even begin. This was the path so many of my business classmates dreamed of. I had *made it*. But it left me asking, "Now what?"

In hindsight, I am not sure if many, or any, of these achievements were the result of my own authentic dreams. I enjoyed the process, and I liked some of the "hygiene factors" that came along with them, like prestige, respect, experiences, and compensation, but I certainly took none of these steps purposefully in an attempt to find my true calling.

Despite facing very poor odds of survival, I take great solace in finally having a clearer purpose with a richer and less biased understanding of what I most cherish and what some of my own dreams really are. I also developed a deeper awareness of how intensely personal and idiosyncratic our true purpose really is.

Questions to Ponder as You Shift to Fast Forward:

- Are you currently doing what you were meant to do? Do your professional and personal roles give you great purpose?
- If not, are there aspects of those roles that give you purpose?

Your Professional Purpose

There is often a big difference between what brings money and what brings joy. A professional role that brings a lot of money may not bring stimulating work, responsibility, recognition, or the opportunity for personal growth and development. It may require you to work in a bad *culture*. If you do not enjoy your work, a higher salary is not likely to satisfy your need for fulfillment. You should find happiness in the work itself, not merely the economic or reputation benefits.

Happiness and excellence are closely related, and the pursuit of excellence is a productive and probable path to happiness. Your professional purpose will almost certainly be something you excel in. Carrying out your professional purpose, therefore, is not only rewarding for you and your well-being but also valuable to everyone around you. As Eric Greitens said: "Nobility in work lies not so much in the work that we do but in the excellence we bring to it."

Somewhere near the intersection of money, excellence, and happiness, you'll find your professional purpose, like the sweet spot of a Venn Diagram. Your work really can be meaningful and impactful and can offer you a chance to develop and grow personally while providing an opportunity for ongoing achievement. The hard part is finding or creating the right conditions for you to thrive.

In the pursuit of your professional purpose, you should consider and balance your current aspirations—what you already believe your professional purpose should look like—with emergent opportunities presented throughout your career. Experimentation and discovery are necessary to find the best paths through life.

Additionally, genuine hard work is often required in your professional life and does not, in and of itself, mean a career path is inconsistent with your purpose. The difference between hard work in pursuit of your calling and hard work for less productive ends is that the former will be well worth the time and effort and leave you with a feeling of joy and accomplishment.

A concept associated with work and purpose is *impact*. Impact means something a little different for everyone. I define it as actions resulting in or affecting an outcome that provides inspiration and motivation. While impact often has an obvious influence on others, the more important element is the benefit it presents to you.

Regardless of how you define it, when you can make a big impact on others with your work, your work and career are likely transforming you into the person you aspire to be.

Questions to Ponder as You Shift to Fast Forward:

- What do you love about the work you do?
- What are you uniquely capable of doing?

Your Personal Purpose

Your personal and professional purposes are closely connected. However, most people have important personal priorities that have no relation to their professional ones.

Your personal purpose may be focused more internally—like spending time reading, writing, or exercising—or externally, like providing mentorship, advocacy, or philanthropy. Like your professional purpose, your personal calling should be something you love and excel at. It certainly need not be just one thing. It will also provide you with an opportunity to develop and continue to improve, helping you evolve into the person you desire to be. According to Viktor Frankl, mental health is based on a certain degree of tension: between what one has achieved and what one ought to accomplish, between what one is and what one should become.

I gained more clarity in my personal purpose after my terminal diagnosis. For example, I realized how important it was to me to be a father. I knew I wanted to have children but had no real urgency to make it happen. Fortunately, my incredible and maternalistic wife had long been ready to have kids, and we were able to move quickly after my revelation.

I may run out of time before I get to be a dad, but I can clearly see how important it is to my wife and me, and I will be forever grateful for any day I get to spend in that role. I also understand that having a child will give my wife some version of *me,* as part of a unique combination of *us*—fulfilling her personal aspiration as well.

With the deterioration of my health, writing and sharing my thoughts became imperative. I hope to inspire my friends and family as well as others I may never meet. I want to extract something positive out of something terrible and give others the confidence to do the same.

Questions to Ponder as You Shift to Fast Forward:

- How big an impact have you had on your family, friends, and community?
- How would your closest friends or family members define your personal purpose or calling?

8
Accepting Support

*In the beginning of life, when we are infants,
we need others to survive.
At the end of life, when you get like me,
you need others to survive. But here's the secret:
in between, we need others too.*

—Morrie Schwartz

Physiotherapists and occupational therapists know the importance of consistent back, knee, wrist, and ankle support. Professional athletes and business leaders understand the power of encouraging teammates and colleagues. Many sick or traumatized children benefit greatly from emotional support animals and support groups. And you have likely known the power of having a close and trusted friend when you really needed them. For life's most serious challenges, the expertise of psychiatrists, psychologists, and social workers is sometimes underappreciated. Still, support from others is something we think we do not need very often.

Prior to my original cancer diagnosis, like most people, I had never spoken with a psychiatrist, nor had I ever had a conversation about my mental health with any other professional. I assumed these people were good at their jobs, but not something I needed. I also assumed interactions with these professionals would be forced and unnatural. Though intermittently aware of my stress, usually during periods of severe sleep deprivation and work pressure early in my career, I never took my mental health very seriously.

As part of my initial treatment process, I was assigned both a psychiatrist and a social worker. The topic of mental health also began to frequently surface with my oncologist and primary care physician. I learned quite quickly the essential role of these caring people, especially in challenging situations like mine. To fully accept a significant personal issue, you need to be able to speak in an unbridled and unfiltered way, not trying to protect your listener from your burdens. For their sake and yours, friends and family may not be the best participants in these conversations. With that said, throughout my two cancer fights, I developed a deep gratitude for the support and companionship I received from my wonderful group of friends and family.

I am *not* trying to diagnose mental health issues that are not there. I *am* trying to soften negative stereotypes about receiving professional help and explain the many ways such support—both professional and informal—can improve your well-being. If mental health topics are a bit uncomfortable for you, I hope you will approach this section with an open mind.

Questions to Ponder as You Shift to Fast Forward:

- When have you recommended support for someone you cared about who was going through a challenging time?
- How long would you avoid seeking assistance if you knew it would positively impact your life?

Calling in Professional Reinforcements

If you think you need help mentally or emotionally, even if you feel it's minor, seek it out. Speaking with and benefiting from physicians, often your family doctor first and then a psychiatrist or other mental health professional, is simply a matter of making the first appointment. These individuals have a wealth of experience with patients going through similar situations to yours. As with any interpersonal relationship, it is important to find the right fit between psychotherapy professional and patient, understanding that each practitioner has their own unique style and personality.

With the right professional, you will be able to openly express your feelings and concerns without worrying about being judged or burdening an unprepared listener with your pain or suffering. A trusted professional should also provide thoughtful questions and perspectives and listen attentively as you verbalize and consequently better understand your various concerns and aspirations. They know when to ask a question to get you to go a little deeper on a topic, and they know when to mirror your emotions. For example, they may stop you when you choke up while speaking about a particular person or event, understanding the significance of those emotions.

In my experience, a good psychiatrist is a tremendous gift. These professionals simply want to listen to help improve your mental health. It is amazing how much is on your mind when you are willing to express it. These professionals are helpful even when your mind and emotions are already in a relatively good space. It's important to feel comfortable releasing your emotions in a healthy and unrestrained way. For me, there is no better way to express and understand my feelings than by speaking to a talented psychiatrist or psychologist. Without this venue, your emotions may flare up in an unhealthy way, whether while you are alone or with a close friend or loved one. Properly expressing your emotions and not repressing them, has significant, positive health ramifications. A clear and healthy mind is a powerful thing that requires hard work, including support from the right resources.

Questions to Ponder as You Shift to Fast Forward:

- How comfortable are you with expressing your emotions?
- Is there a challenge in your life that a professional could help you address?

Nurturing Your Key Personal Relationships

You should invest in your most important personal relationships years before you need anything from them in return. Love and unconditional support come from long-tenured, genuine, mutually beneficial relationships. The best, most durable relationships I have are founded on dependability, mutual respect, shared values, and a focus on each other's growth and development.

As I have mentioned before, phone calls, coffees, lunches, and dinners with your closest friends are the connections that build long, durable bonds. Both parties benefit from the comradery, companionship, and fellowship that naturally occurs in the process. "I'm busy" is no excuse to deprioritize your most important relationships. By genuinely and sincerely investing in these friendships early and often, you build reserves of emotional support for the future.

Prior to my diagnosis, I wasn't a very trusting person. I tended to take care of myself and not ask for much help; however, I discovered the unconditional support poured out from my most important relationships had extraordinary power to positively influence my response to and recovery from unfortunate events in my life. This encouragement increased my confidence and comfort through a number of challenging situations. Throughout my two cancer fights, I benefitted tremendously from my personal support structure. I had no idea how much I would need these people when we invested time in them years ago. As Clay Christensen said, "You can't plant saplings when you need the shade of a tall tree."

Questions to Ponder as You Shift to Fast Forward:

- What characteristics are consistent across your very best relationships?
- How often do you think of the health of your most important relationships?
- How hard would you be willing to work to avoid losing a relationship with someone who is deeply important to you?

Finding the Right Role Models

We think of children as being highly impressionable, but I believe adults are impressionable too. We are highly influenced by those around us. Therefore, choose to spend time with extraordinary people—those who exhibit the traits you want in your life. The corollary is we should also unapologetically free ourselves from people who are bad for us and our development. These people bring out our worst and hold us back from becoming the people we want to be.

Your closest friends and mentors are likely your most powerful role models. You may also have external role models you have never met. Some of my external role models include Morrie Schwartz, for his ability to face critical illness with grace; Derek Jeter, with both his skill and professionalism as an athlete and his philanthropic work; Charlie Munger, for his wisdom; and Hans Rosling, for his clear vision and unflinching optimism. Some of my personal role models include my parents, my late paternal grandfather, my current boss, my best friends, and my wife. These people have collectively taught me to be open to change, reasonable, generous, devoted to my family, and a good friend, as well as aspire to get better every day, be a great partner, have empathy, and be fearless in the face of adversity.

I am sure many people in your life are happy to provide you with advice, perhaps too often of the unsolicited variety. As you know, not all advice has to be accepted and applied. When you do need advice, solicit it from your most trusted advisors and personal role models. The best counselors wait to be asked but do not hold back their advice when requested.

Your role models do not need to demonstrate exemplary behavior across every aspect of their lives. Nobody is flawless, and you can choose which of your mentors' traits to embody. Even your dog can teach you important lessons—like loyalty and living in the present—but you probably do not need to spin around four times before you lay down.

Questions to Ponder as You Shift to Fast Forward:

- Who have been your most important role models?
- Who do you rely on for advice in difficult situations?

9

Conclusion

As I wrote the preceding pages, I became aware of some themes that were consistent throughout my experience. The following ideas made the most impact on my fast-forward life.

Staying Relentlessly Present

If I learned anything from this process, it is that you can only really address the issues you currently face, one by one, in the present. There is very little you can do to stop or change the challenges you face down the road. For example, I do not allow myself to think about passing away and the likely painful, unknowable process of dying over a period of days, weeks, or months. This process will come, it will be immensely challenging, and I hope to confront it in the moment with courage and grace. But I can do virtually nothing today to alleviate that eventual pain and suffering. I am far better off focusing on today's challenges and opportunities than dwelling on an unknown, potentially horrifying future. I do not hide from this eventual reality, but I intentionally elect to focus my energy more productively for the time being.

Another important realization for me was that in death, I am losing the same thing others lose when they die—life, family, and friends. When I began processing my impending mortality, my first instincts caused me to believe I somehow would lose more than others. The main difference between me and others is simply my age—I will lose these things earlier than most. If you tend to plan or think long-term, the challenge of staying in the moment is likely an even bigger obstacle for you. We must consciously and proactively work to stay in the here and now. We cannot control events that may be weeks and months down the road.

Being relentlessly present is especially important when life shifts into fast forward. Impending death provides you with tension, clarity, and urgency. When doctors put a number on your days, it compounds the need to stay present and properly experience joy and purpose. With fewer and fewer chances to correct mistakes, we have to look for opportunities to bring joy and purpose to others. I do not believe knowing the end is close makes it easier to stay present, but it certainly makes it more important. Additionally, the present is the only place where you are able to keep your mind and body in the right place to fight.

As a relatively young person, it is strange to know the approximate amount of time you have left, especially when it is not very long. The classic dilemma, "How would you live your last days if you knew which day was going to be your last?" has become my reality. I want to use my last days to spend time with the people I love, enjoy beautiful bodies of water, play golf, and start a family with my wife.

Never Giving Up

After receiving my original cancer diagnosis and learning the severity and need for chemotherapy, radiation, and surgery, I spoke with a number of former cancer patients and read various information packages to better understand treatment side effects.

About nine months after my original diagnosis, after completing chemotherapy, radiation, and surgery, doctors deemed me cancer-free. I spent five months back to normal before receiving my recurrence diagnosis and terminal prognosis. At that point, I accepted the day would likely come when I would feel completely beaten down physically. I refused, however, to accept becoming beaten down mentally, and I promised my loved ones that I would never stop fighting, no matter what happened. Though physical defeat seemed inevitable, I refused to be defeated mentally.

While it may sound egotistical, I would love to be one of the most inspiring people my wife, friends, and family have ever known. Being this kind of person would mean the world to me because it would imply I had positively and profoundly impacted them. As a non-religious person, my only hope for carrying on after I die is through the indelibility of the impressions I made on the people around me. I hope that by showing resilience, determination, and strength through the most challenging circumstances and by simply never giving up, I am worthy of even a part of this honor. Even in my darkest moments, I seek to eradicate any feelings of defeat or complacency to continue to challenge and push myself to grow and learn. I am incredibly fortunate to have my family, friends, and physicians. They have made a tremendous difference in holding me up, and they constantly remind me why I refuse to give up.

I am aware that the pain and discomfort associated with my critical illness is likely to increase as time passes.

Unfortunately, I have already experienced this transition. I am also aware that the intensifying disease will likely make it harder for me to continue to fight and make me want to give up. Understanding this dynamic gives me a better appreciation for it each day. However, I owe it to too many people, myself included, not to give up. These people deserve an unrelenting fight until my very last day on Earth.

Never Growing Old

After I was first diagnosed with my terminal illness, I found myself fantasizing about living a long, happy life. While doing so, I never dreamed of growing old. I was certainly comfortable with the idea of adding another candle to my birthday cake each year and, hopefully, growing wiser and more mature. I was less enthralled with the part of aging that includes aches and pains, exercising and traveling less, and seeking out fewer new opportunities.

As I said at the beginning of this book, we are all in the business of living, not dying. When you are in a position like mine, you develop a special appreciation for staying youthful, energetic, and curious. Regardless of my situation, I want to continue to live my life fully. I want to soak up the sunshine and the warmth of the people I love. I also aspire to continue to learn and grow. As one of my excellent physicians said, "Younger patients who are very sick tend to keep on living, and then, one day, they die; with older patients, they often start the process of dying well before they die."

I believe adventure is an important part of a full and rewarding life. However, as we age or get very sick, we tend to shy away from adventure. Personally, I do not believe energy and curiosity are necessarily impacted by our remaining longevity. If we keep pushing ourselves outside our comfort zones, we will continue to grow—even as we age. There is beauty in living a youthful, active, and healthy lifestyle. Even if you expect to live beyond ninety, you do not need to grow old. I've seen many beautiful examples of mothers and fathers actively and energetically participating in the lives of their adult children, grandchildren, and even great-grandchildren. They become caregivers, have fun, and act as mentors. Of course, age is more than just a number; but it does not need to be.

Losing Your Self

One of the most fundamental psychological changes that happened to me after becoming terminally ill was the realization that everything was not really about me anymore—as if it ever had been. My life quickly became more about the people I loved and the people I could help through writing about my experiences and sharing my perspectives. Losing my "self" in this process was certainly not a bad thing. It gave me greater clarity of vision and purpose. Focusing externally instead of internally made it easier for me to listen and be empathetic, patient, and quiet. The realization that your life is no longer about you is also a very good reminder of who you are fighting for and, therefore, why you refuse to stop.

The concept of "self" can be pretty convoluted. It has been broadly discussed in psychology, philosophy, and religious circles. The idea of self and not-self is discussed in depth in Buddhist and meditation literature. I had loosely practiced meditation in the years leading up to my terminal diagnosis. After my recurrence, however, I started meditating in a more deliberate way. I believed in the essence and possibility of self-transcendence—moving beyond self and realizing it is a fictitious thing—but assumed I would never experience the state. Everyone can benefit from periodically asking, "Is life really all about me?" Though the answer is "of course not," it wasn't until I became critically ill that I truly understood this truth for myself. I will still not claim that I have obtained self-transcendence; however, I have become less focused on myself, and I feel very grateful for this change.

Saying Good-Bye

When I first heard that my cancer had returned and was incurable, I thought I had one silver lining. I would never have to see the people I love get sick, gradually decline, and ultimately pass away—perhaps avoiding a lot of very painful goodbyes. I quickly realized, however, that I would still need to say all the goodbyes and likely many more. And I would need to do so over a much shorter time period.

While difficult and traumatizing, having the opportunity to say good-bye to the people I love, with the time and capacity to do so thoughtfully, has been a privilege I am genuinely grateful for. I hope to also use the process of saying my goodbyes as a way of putting the people in my life at some level of ease before I go.

This book is giving me an additional way to say goodbye to my loved ones, and the many people I hope will benefit from my story. I will say goodbye by spending time with the people I love and telling them about their importance in my life. This opportunity has helped me become a little more at ease with the idea of leaving them once and for all.

Epilogue

Amanda Hammond Gray

On March 31, 2020, my husband and the author of this book, James J. Hammond, passed away at the age of twenty-eight. Despite his diagnosis and prognosis, James's death came quite unexpectedly. In the midst of some very routine appointments at the hospital—his weekly transfusions and his twelfth lung tap—his heart stopped. Due to the strict lockdowns of the COVID-19 pandemic, the hospital kept visitors and caregivers to a minimum. So, this was the first time I was unable to attend his appointments with him.

    I have replayed this day over and over in my head a thousand times. I dropped him off at Princess Margaret Cancer Center, kissed him goodbye, and told him I would see him in a few hours when he was done. He walked into the hospital independently; I had absolutely no reason for concern. After the nurse called to tell me he had collapsed but was conscious and being monitored closely, I made my way to the hospital without a second thought for the no-visitor restrictions that would greet me when I arrived. I was driving along University Avenue with the hospital in view when I received the call telling me James had suddenly died.

I have never experienced pain like that of losing James. I disagree wholeheartedly with his statement that "the pain goes away." It has certainly *changed* as time has passed, but the ache is still just as raw and real as the day he died. When memories from that horrible day creep back into my mind, it almost feels like a movie, as if it didn't actually happen to us. Sometimes, I still cannot believe he isn't here. I can still hear his voice in my head, and whenever I need advice, he is the first person I ask. It's funny how our brain plays tricks on us. Almost immediately after he died, I pictured him as a healthy 26-year-old man whenever I recalled memories. Even if I was thinking of something he said the week before his death, I conveniently blocked the sickness, the fragility, the cancer. He was just James—healthy, full of life, wise beyond his years, loving and selfless for his people, my first and forever love. There is something beautiful about this protective barrier my brain has created, as James is truly forever young in my memories. However, his death has given me an even greater appreciation for birthdays and aging, and I will endlessly wish he was growing older right alongside me.

From the time we were teenagers, James and I had plans to raise a family and grow old together. At the time of his death, I was four months pregnant with our son. This beautiful boy is truly the light of our lives. I feel immense joy that James's son has this book to get to know his father and see how brave, intelligent, resilient, loving, and inspiring he was.

If you had the pleasure of meeting or knowing James, I hope reading this book opened a window into his beautiful mind and made you smile to hear his voice in these pages. If you have never met James, I feel privileged to have given you a glimpse of the most amazing person I have ever known, loved, and lost.

Meet James Hammond

James grew up in London, Ontario and lived most recently in the Beaches neighborhood of Toronto with his wife, Amanda, and their Bernese Mountain Dog, Harvin.

He attended Western University and received an Honors Bachelor of Arts in Business Administration (with distinction) at the Ivey Business School as well as an Honors Bachelor of Science in Actuarial Science (also with distinction). James became an Associate of both the Society of Actuaries and the Canadian Institute of Actuaries.

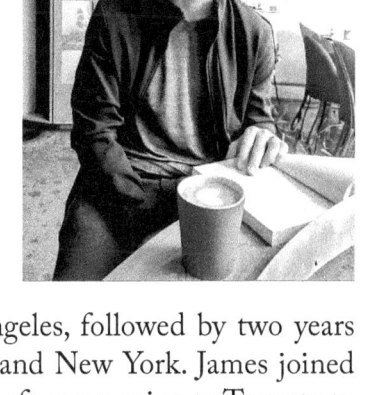

James completed two summer internships in investment banking at Barclays in Los Angeles, followed by two years at Goldman Sachs in Toronto and New York. James joined TPG Capital in San Francisco before returning to Toronto to continue his private equity career at Altas Partners. James also co-founded and chaired the board of a Canadian charitable foundation focused on supporting underprivileged youth athletes across Ontario.

James was first diagnosed with cancer just a few months after returning to Toronto from San Francisco. His tumor was identified as Alveolar Rhabdomyosarcoma (A-RMS), a rare and often lethal form of pediatric sarcoma, which was localized in his right forearm. James received a treatment regimen at Princess Margaret Cancer Centre that included nine months of chemotherapy, one month of radiation therapy, and surgery. After these treatments, he was deemed "cancer-free," returning to his routine of hard work, exercise, and spending time with friends and family, along with a new appreciation for life's ups and downs.

Unfortunately, a few weeks before his twenty-eighth birthday, James's cancer returned. The disease had spread throughout much of his body, and James was informed that it was likely incurable. Over the following six months, James completed eight one-week cycles of intensive chemotherapy—seven cycles before his cancer overcame the first regimen and one cycle before it overcame the second regimen. With conventional treatments failing, James elected to enter an A-RMS clinical trial based at the National Institutes of Health in Bethesda, Maryland. James's cancer overcame the protocol after two months of treatment. Consequently, James restarted chemotherapy and radiotherapy treatment in Toronto to try to manage his progressing disease. Tragically, following a routine procedure, he went into cardiac arrest and could not be resuscitated.

The James J. Hammond Fund was established to positively impact many future patients facing similarly dire situations and, ultimately, offer them a cure. See jjhfund.org for more information.

Credits and Book Recommendations

Below is a collection of the most thoughtful and life-changing books I have ever read. Many of these books shaped the way I think about the world and the person I have become. To these incredible authors and for their experiences and challenges, I am forever grateful.

1. *Man's Search for Meaning* by Victor Frankl
2. *The Wisdom of Insecurity* by Alan Watts
3. *Tuesdays with Morrie* by Mitch Albom
4. *How Will You Measure Your Life* by Clay Christensen
5. *Resilience* by Eric Greitens
6. *Meditations* by Marcus Aurelius
7. *12 Rules for Life* by Jordan B. Peterson
8. *Influence* by Robert Cialdini
9. *How to Win Friends & Influence People* by Dale Carnegie
10. *Poor Charlie's Almanack* by Charlie Munger

Personal Notes

www.ingramcontent.com/pod-product-compliance
Lightning Source LLC
Chambersburg PA
CBHW050225100526
44585CB00017BA/2051